75 THINGS I *HATE* ABOUT BEING HANDICAPPED

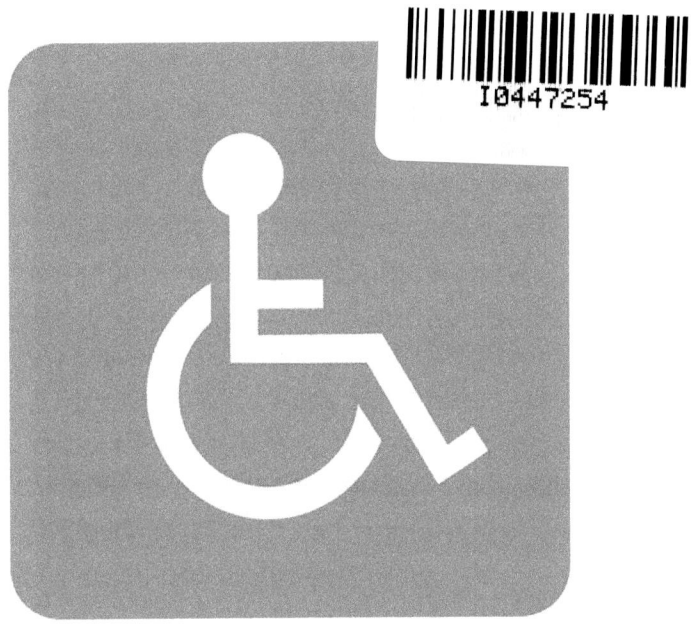

I0447254

75 THINGS I *LIKE* ABOUT BEING HANDICAPPED

BY: B.S. KNOT

Where I'm sure that the following 150 *things* will raise some eye brows. I can hear some already saying to just deal with your handicap, accept it because there's nothing you can do about it so just get on with your life. As an individual approaching 50 years of age and being handicap my entire life, I'm fully capable of deciding for myself whether I enjoy being handicap or if I accept it. I have decades of experience in these manners. One of my best friends also had muscular dystrophy and he totally accepted it, he was completely comfortable in his own skin. I'm not like that, I'm no different than a normal person who doesn't like the way they look. Where some opt for plastic surgery, breast augmentation, liposuction... there is no operation for some handicap people. I am imprisoned in this bent, broken, crooked, deformed body for life. I'm entitled to posses my own opinions and disappointments. Just because I have a physical handicap does not provide the right of others to dictate my thoughts or feelings.

HATE

1) I hate being manhandled… I get that you're bigger and stronger than I am, but is your self esteem so low that you need to slap, shake or pin a handicap person?

2) Don't ask "what's *wrong* with you?" It's impolite and frankly none of your business. If we become friends, I'll discuss it with you at a later time. Do you walk up to complete strangers and ask how much money is in their bank account. No, it is not an acceptable behavior. So, please reserve your inquisition until we are acquainted.

3) Yes, I know, I look different than other people, but as a kid I hated being starred at like I was a touring member of the freak show and now decades later, I'm just

sick and tired of being starred at.

4) My arms do not extend beyond a 90 degree angle and I'm 5 foot 5 inches tall which of course means everything I ever want to purchase is inevitably located on a top shelf beyond my reach. Of course it never fails as I stare at the A1 Steak Sauce or the Smoked Chipotle Tabasco, trying to somehow levitate upwards and because there seems to be some kind of intergalactic power design to further humiliate me, but every time I stop to stare at the top shelf product, a 4 foot 10 inch grandmother approaches and asks if I can please grab her a bottle of Hellman's 1000 Island Dressing from the top shelf? It never gets any easier replying, "no, I'm sorry I can't". Nobody likes that evil grandma look designed to let you know she thinks you're a jackass. My nature however is to be

helpful, so I'd grab it if I could, I just can't grams. I've also yet to figure out why everyone else in the world seems to immediately recognize I have a handicap *except* grandma's measuring in at under 5 feet in height.

5) While on the subject of my arm's inabilities to extend beyond an L shape, here's a few more reasons I hate being handicapped. Starting with my feet… clipping my toe nails is a hootin' good time. Just bending and reaching that far is a major obstacle, but I have very limited dexterity in my hands and fingers so bending, reaching and clipping tends to be a scheduled morning affair. Where most people accomplish this feat in minutes, it takes me minimally an hour of stretching, flexing, twisting, manipulating and grunting.

6) I can't reach my back pocket so I don't carry a wallet. I carry bare essentials in a shirt pocket; driver's license, a credit/debit card and a small amount of cash. You certainly don't want to carry any significant amount of cash when it is exposed to the public. Shirts are generally limited to button down shirts. Very rarely do you find polo, t-shirts, sweat shirts, sweaters or anything of a pull over design having a pocket. I'd like to dress more fashionable or even more causally on occasion, but my handicap dictates my wardrobe.

7) I don't put things in my front pant pocket either. Because of the limited extension or reach, lack of dexterity, I appear to be playing pocket pool if I'm digging in my pocket trying to retrieve the desired object.

8) I can't reach the back of the refrigerator, so never, ever eat

anything from the back while visiting. IT AIN"T FRESH!!!

9) I can't do drive-thru services. I can't reach far enough to hand over, pay, receive or conduct any type of transaction.

10) My lack of reach and need for wearing dress shirts results in a using a tool to tuck the shirt into my pants. I utilize an 18" long metal shoe horn to dress on a daily basis. A public need to use a restroom results in my shirt not returning to a quality tuck or being tucked at all.

11) With bathrooms in mind, I never use urinals. Because I have to bend over so far to reach my waistline coupled with my short stature, it essentially puts my face in the urinal. On the rare occasion I am forced to use a urinal, my stance frequently leads to obnoxious

comments, unwelcomed stares and unpleasant results.

12) Anything located on the ground becomes a debate on whether it is worth the difficulty in retrieving it. Where most people just bend over to pick it up, I lack that ability. I simply cannot reach that far. If I need to pick anything up off the ground I must kneel to my right knee and then try and scoop it up. Because of the lack of dexterity coins make a quandary in regards to effort. I don't even consider picking up pennies, nickels or dimes… it's just not worth the effort or the entertainment value I provide others. Quarters up require the scanning of how many I'll entertain. The worst place to drop anything on the ground is while in line at a retail outlet. Those in line have nothing else to do than watch as I struggle to collect my dropped item. I've had children act as if they were going

to kick me in the ass as I hunched over trying to pry something of the floor which brought no reaction for the moron mothers.

13) I tie my shoes while sitting in a chair by crossing my leg, ankle to a knee. If a shoe comes untied while in public, it stays untied. It's not overly common to have chairs in the potato chip isle, paint row or meat market. I can't kneel and tie my shoes, but I do appreciate the stares and comments, "don't that boy know his shoe is untied?"

14) While on the name calling… I get I'm small and frail looking, but when you call me "Big Guy" don't get upset when I reply back with "Slim" or "Einstein". If we're greeting each other in terms of opposites and I'm not supposed to be insulted with "Big Guy" then take no offense to being called "Slim". Were just sharing terms of endearment right?

15) In terms of greeting... I can't help I can't shake your hand, I want to, they just don't work. I try to ignore the request of a hand shake as much as possible but my conscious demands I extend what constitutes or is equivalent to a recently deceased calamari. It would have been easier for me if I had been born in an Asian area of the world where we could just bow, but I guess if I was granted a wish it wouldn't be a relocation or culture of birth.

16) Yes, I have useless hands. They say the difference between man and other animals is thumbs. I am not an animal! But my thumbs do not extend, there is no opening them for a handshake as mentioned, or any other function. My fingers are pretty much non functioning too so the following is a list of *things I hate* regarding my hands or lack of dexterity.

17) I can't hitchhike… without the ability to raise my thumb, to passing motorist I simply look like a cripple guy standing along the side of the road waving a partial fist as they pass by.

18) I cannot point… my hands have an arthritic appearance, my index finger does not go straight, it does not operate independently of the other fingers, well frankly it just doesn't function and with the existence of a curve, everyone would be looking off or following directions to the left even though I meant to go straight forward.

19) There's no peace sign coming from these hands. It may be old school, but it's my school and I'd like to flash a peace sign periodically.

20) Couldn't ever join a gang, I couldn't do all that hand gesturing those folks do. I suppose I could start my own gang "The Crips" and a bunch of us cripple people could terrorize the citizens, but I highly doubt our hand signs would actually be exact... more like, again, a gang thrusting out a recently deceased calamari.

21) A personal heavy hearted limitation... I cannot flip people off. Granted it may prevent repeated beatings, but bouts of road rage where I try and give someone the bird only results in continued torment as the offending driver is now laughing hysterically at my calamari.

22) I cannot pick up a glass, I have to use both hands and essentially mash my hands together to lift it to my mouth. I have found this to be surprising an ANTI-Aphrodisiac. Sort of like drinking with Flipper or a trained seal. "Honk the horn B.S., we'll toss you a sardine!"

23) A few other things most take for granted; I cannot use scissors ~ nope! Don't have the extension of my thumbs. There is no opening of scissors or an ability to cut.

24) Tweezers; limited dexterity equals limited use.

25) Tongs don't work either so salad bars or buffets don't appeal to me.

26) Buffets also present the trouble of my lack of arm extension. My face is generally plastered against the glass germ guard to begin with but a dish located against a wall or the other side of the buffet, unless I want to endure the wrath of dirty looks for actually ducking under or inside the buffet, I can only go home hoping the out of reach tapioca pudding sucked.

27) I can't clap. With two calamaris as hands the sound much more resembles a faint phwap phwap

sound. Please forgive me if I just nod in improvement.

28) High five is out. No arm extension and who really wants to slap a squid?

29) You ladies are safe from a tender swat on your behind. With a need to slightly bend at the waist and a nonfunctioning hand applied to the derriere, it becomes much less affectionate and far more a moment of "what the…"

30) Can't dribble

31) Can't bowl

32) Can't put on a baseball glove

33) Another personal torment is I can't operate hand brakes on bicycles or motorcycles. I'd love to be able to ride a motorcycle but within the first 1000 yards the motorbike would evolve into B.S.'s mode death.

34) I guess it's ok I can't ride a motorcycle because I couldn't maintain it. It is very difficult for me to put a nut onto a bolt. If it's at a weird angle and in need of threading, 90 percent of the time the nut will be flung out into the yard.

35) I look really stupid riding bikes anyways. With my arms at 90 degrees, it's not like I look good or normal on bike to begin with. Most comfortable bike I ever rode was my childhood banana seat Columbia with long handlebars.

36) Continuing with the dexterity deficiencies of my life… I can't play piano. Bummer

37) I can't play the guitar. Bigger bummer

38) I no longer can play drums. A huge bummer. I used to play and loved playing, but even in my youth I dropped a lot of sticks and now my

fingers are way too weak to run around a set. I had a beautiful black Premier Resonator set that I sat behind for hours upon hours. The dream of being the next Keith Moon has long gone but I still recall with great fondness playing in Matt's back yard, at parties in the shed and my worst performance atop a flat bed trailer when the weather was frigid and I could barely hold a stick to play. Great memories those days brought and remain with me, but scoring chicks through musical aptitude has passed.

39) What else can't my hands do? Well I don't open bottles with my hands, I use my teeth to most people's chagrin. Plastic bottles generally get a little look of concern, but opening a twist off beer bottle causes most to look with great amazement, or perplexity.

40) Without an open, flat hand, 90 percent of the time change misses its target. At the checkout line I generally get my change in portions. The first pouring, followed by the clerk scooping up the coins that missed and occasionally a final pouring of any that missed the first, second, third… to a final portion. Yep, I generally use a debit card!

41) I can't run, so I'm ideal to camp near bears with. With the old adage, "all I have to do is out run you!" pretty much leaves me to the wolves, bears and muggers.

42) Obviously I don't camp much.

43) And I was always picked last in gym.

44) In fact, I'm generally picked last for everything. I play euchre with great skills ~ last. I do trivia games well ~ last. Darts~ well I'd pick myself last too!

45) I do seem to always be the first in one category... blame. "Who used my wife's hand towels Knot!" "Well it wasn't me." "Who caused my stocks to drop you SOB?" "Dad, how the heck could impact the stock market?" "Who drank the last beer?" "ummm well that one is on me"

46) I HATE those that mimic my deformities. It is NOT funny. No one in blackface is funny. No one acting Asian by pulling at their eyes is funny. Wanna make fun of my clothes? Fine! I chose and put them on in the morning, but my physical appearance is mental burden on me which I do not like. I do not want to look like this! It is not funny whether I know you, whether you're a relative or a narcissistic ex-girlfriend. There is no relationship in the past, present or the future of my life that makes it acceptable to mock something

that cause me constant mental anguish.

47) While we're on things that piss me off. I hate hearing, "at least you have your health". No, I don't. I never did.

48) "I'm just glad my child was born healthy." We all are, but you don't have to apologize to me when you say that.

49) I seem to create great anger in those that deem me smarter than them. I'm not mad at you for being able to run, play basketball, ride a motorcycle, shake someone's hand. I'm not angry at you for being physically superior to me, why such hostility towards me for being mentally superior to you?

50) If you ask me to do something and I try but unable to physically do it, don't rant and rave. I'm already angry with myself, I'm already embarrassed for myself, I'm

already emasculated, so it's not really necessary to further humiliate me. I'm intelligent enough to understand your ranting a raving is a cloaked way of indicating your belief I'm a "worthless cripple". I'd have done it if I could, I certainly didn't want to endure your veiled reference.

51) I hate the day after Labor Day. No you didn't donate money to me over Labor Day. You donated money to the Muscular Dystrophy Association. I have never received a single benefit from them. It's not like they rake it in and then disperse the funds among us to make our lives more comfortable or manageable. If you want to donate money to me, I'll hold out my calamari.

52) It would be nice if the MDA had some type of life preparation, training, educational benefits because I have had my share of

troubles with employment and
educational funds in my life.

53) As previously stated, college
funding was essentially non-
existent to me. Ohio's Vocational
Board of Rehabilitation indicated
in my youth that having muscular
dystrophy with limited physical
abilities did not warrant
assistance.

54) The military however found my
handicap to be worthy of
preventing me from joining in
order to earn college tuition.

55) I side with the military, I wouldn't
have had any business in any
branch. I could climb stairs back
then, but the rope hanging down a
wall to scale was in my world a
giant wick to burn it down and
eventually proceed through the
ashes. Currently, stairs are simply
a jagged wall and they may as well
throw a rope down them.

56) Well I take that back. You put a pretty lady at the top of those stairs and I'll crawl up them. Of course by experience, they always seem to move faster than me. For some reason, dudes with squid hands are not considered worthy of companionship.

57) I got use to the opposite sex finding me repulsive in my youth. Ever have a girl refuse to kiss you while playing spin the bottle? Oh no it's not crushing at all, I mean I barely remember the event on a daily basis.

58) The girl in high school that always said yes said "no way!"

59) Ever open the door and have an escort say "I'm sorry, I got the wrong address" while scurrying down the walk way. Ummm, me neither.

60) What other humiliating thing do I hate that I can relay to you. Oh, I

hate button down fly jeans. It's not so much that I hate the pants themselves, it's just that I can't wear them because of my inability to button them. So just don't buy them you may say. I don't, but like clockwork when I still received birthday and Christmas gifts from my parents, I was gifted them. I'd open the box and walla, button down fly Levi's. "Mom you know I can't wear button down fly jeans, how many times do I have to tell you this?" "Oh, I'll exchange them." 2 months later on Christmas and SURPRISE, same damn pants. "It's not the gift but the thought that counts", says mom. Hmmm, a painful reoccurrence twice a year, yes mom, very thoughtful. Thank you ever so much.

61) Speaking of parenting, I hate that I will never have children. I feel robbed that I'll never know the joy seeing my child being born, going off the school, growing into

adulthood and reveling in their success. And I'm thoroughly disappointed in the fact I'll never be able to buy them button down fly jeans twice a year.

62) Yes, I'm physically capable of having offspring. Two things however prevent me from having children; one ~ I choose in high school that I would not have a child, that I didn't wish to pass this gene on and have another person live the hell that is my life. Two ~ it requires a female partner and apparently while I was making a conscious decision not to have children, the women of the world were conspiring and amending the "Woman's Manual" to also prevent a Knot kid. Their amendment has been amazingly successful.

63) Which brings me to another hate my handicap brings; isolation and loneliness. I so violate the commandment of envy, because I

envy those with companionship immensely. The daily conversations, spending holidays with someone, having someone to spoil and compliment. I did have a short taste, I did live with a girl for awhile but it became apparent quickly that I was less a companion and more a lap dog. When she felt like petting me on the head, I was worthy of attention and the rest of the 167 and half hours of the week, I was treated as if I soiled the rug. I didn't clean the stove right, I didn't load the dishwasher right, I didn't clean the bathroom right, 4 nights a week of cooking was not enough, I raked the leaves in a pile in the wrong spot, I wasn't a real drummer, I was an embarrassment in public so I was left home, when she wanted to go to bed she got up, turned the television off, lights out and left me sitting in the dark. My absolute favorite part of living with her was when she left a lamp on and I tried to turn it off but my calamari couldn't twist the switch. I endured a lovely emasculating beat down for her lit lamp. I had high hopes of a companion and friendship and in the end she wasn't even friendly. Well I'm a big time sinner folks, because I am so envious of all of you that have a life partner.

64) I hate having to ask someone to take the cap off an ink pen.

65) I hate watching others with less credentials being promoted over me.

66) I hate that I don't have the strength to drive a classic car. Love the lines of cars built in the 40's 50's and 60's but I tried to drive a buddy's classic Mustang once. I wasn't strong enough to mash the clutch down and no power

steering means the car is going wherever it's pointed.

67) I hate the fact with two squids for hands, placing a nail and attempting to drive it in provides for mashed calamari served with profanity.

68) Oh, here's one I hate. Because of the lack of arm extension when I clean a toilet bowl my face is far too close to gross surfaces. I really need a biohazard face shield for this necessary evil activity.

69) Where most people take opening things for granted, I struggle with: jars, potato chip bags, zip lock bags, childproof caps, Fed Ex bags, CANS!!!, don't hand me a manual can opener. Want to keep me out of a room, put one of those child proof door knob thingy's on it and then I won't be able to open the door.

70) I hate that there are limited jobs available for me. I feel like I'm a hard hat and work boot dude in a broken little buddy. I want to drive a crane, frame a house, captain a fishing boat... but in reality, I've never been who I wanted to be.

71) I hate I can't flick a booger

72) Or use a bar of soap. Liquid soap for calamari boy.

73) I hate I can't pick up anything over 50 pounds, which explains why I can't pick up chicks.

74) I hate the way the world looks at me.

75) And I hate that I truly like my character, I know I'm a good person who always thinks of others first. (Which frequently leads to being taken advantage of.) I like the fact I have intelligence, humor and compassion. Makes it all more conflicting when I can

honestly say I hate being me. I've hated being me every day of my life. There is not a day that goes by where I'm not reminded personally or by others that I'm unable, incapable, unworthy, unbecoming, unattractive, unacceptable, inept, unhappy, unappreciated, unemployed, undesirable, intolerable, invisible... With so much alone time, I frequently ponder what life would have been like if I was born with my character, my personality, my intelligence, my soul but with a normal body. It wouldn't have to have been modelesque, just arms, hands, legs that worked... how much different would my life have been? How much happier, fulfilling, rewarding and social activity would there have been? I don't have to be reminded it is what it is, but when your days are filled of thought, you tend to ponder these questions. But as I just said, it is what it is, so on with the things I like about being handicapped.

LIKE

1) I like parking in handicap parking spots. Wait, I don't have a permit, I've never applied for one. Always thought others were more deserving. I really should rethink my stance judging by those I see get out of their cars, the four wheel drive trucks I could never physically get in and the lack of dings they seem to have on the door panels.

2) I like, umm… well I suppose I like… no really don't like that. I'll have a pop tart and see what I can conjure up.

3) My last entry was from a few days back and I have to tell you, I still haven't come up with a like so I'll readdress this again a later date.

4) Week two and nothing, maybe next week.

5) A month on and the May sun has yet to bring up a handicap like. I'll keep working on one.

6) June ~ sorry

7) July ~ nope

8) August and this humidity is brutal. But nothing yet.

9) Hey, wait that's a hate

10) October it's my birthday. No I don't like my birthday, I'd rather I was never born. But I am working on a like.

11) Merry Christmas readers. No I don't like Christmas either. Nowhere to go, no one to spend it with although I am mindful that some years ago it would be time to open a box containing button down fly jeans.

12) Happy New Year... and no.

13) 2007

14) 2008

15) I really would like to get this book done but I'm just not coming up with any likes.

16) Wait, nope, sorry.

17) Nada

18) Rein

19) El mitaan

20) Nichts

21) I like calling my hands calamari, but I don't like my hands. This may be a push.

22) 2009

23) 2010

24) Naught

25) I'm drawing a blank

26) Not a dog gone thing in mind yet.

27) Void of "like" thought

28) I'm open to suggestions

29) I like… ummm… oh come on man, just make one up for Pete's sake.

30) I like nurses! Can we let this one slide as something of an attempt?

31) I've had a 3 week migraine just trying to come up with ONE thing I like but…

32) I like the MDA symbol, but I'd rather not be associated with it.

33) Ohhh I like the fact I remember my sister watching the MDA telephone when Dean Martin came out and surprised Jerry Lewis. I know, I'm clutching at straws but I am truly trying to find something.

34) Ahhh haaa, I got one! I can use it to weasel out of doing things I don't want to do! "I'm sorry I'd like to help you dig a ditch, but I just can't physically do it." Well that's a real relief for me. Several years since the inception of this book

and I finally came up with one. Ok, how many more do I have to go?

35) I like... well let's get to know me. I like warm weather. I don't function well in the cold.

36) I like music, all kinds of music. I grew up on The Beatles, Stones, Who and Zeppelin. Grew into a huge fan of Jimmy Buffett, surf music, calypso music... jazz, an itty little bit of classical. I saw a lot of concerts in my youth with some friends but as they aged and began to go with girlfriends and wives, I was frequently left out. I also got to the point where due to my size and weakness, being anywhere with large crowds was no fun, so I just enjoy tunes on the stereo anymore.

37) I like sports. One of my biggest disappointments in life is I never had the opportunity to participate. I would have liked to try baseball,

maybe football, but I wish now I could golf. Golf I think would have been right up my alley. I love being outside, although your competing against others, your also playing within yourself. Well I feel some anger and disappointment building so I'll try and come up with some likes another day.

38) I like pina coladas

39) And getting caught in the rain (not really to either one but it sounded good at the time)

40) Oh come on there must be something I like about being disabled

41) I just woke from a golden slumber with a like but by the time I got to the computer I had forgot it. Sorry!

42) I'm open to suggestions

43) I gotta goose egg...

44) Wait… wait… wait… nah that ain't one either

45) You have a suggestion… contact me via phone, email, postal, smoke signals or telepathically.

46) I like the Toyota i-REAL personal mobility device, but I doubt I'd ever be able to afford one.

47) Ohh, I think someone is trying to contact me telepathically… hey that's not very friendly. I appreciate everyone's opinions, but I could have done without receiving that.

48) Nil

49) Null

50) Naught

51) Zilch

52) Zippo

53) Well another birthday has past and still nothing… however I did

not receive a pair of button down fly jeans.

54) This may be fringe? I once had some leg braces as a child that had boots made from kangaroo. It gave me no hop, I now feel bad for the kangaroo, but they were an extremely soft leather. Oh, I hated the braces, my mom used to tie the tightest, most evil knots to keep me in them, but they always eventually were solved and the braces discarded in a corner.

55) I like the fact I was unable to become a professional hockey player. Them dudes are bad assed. I did ice skate for a short period of time. My parents were too cheap to buy me a pair of skates so they spray painted a my sisters white skates black and sent me out on the ice. In all fairness, I understand the teasing and beatings I took from the other boys and GIRLS.

56) Here's a quality like! I very much like the fact I'm too short to ride anything other than the tea cups at most amusement parks. Has nothing to do with being handicapped, but it does give me an excuse not to ride roller coasters without saying I'm scared to death of them!

57) Another short like. I like the fact I can wear garanimals. I'd be a fashion nightmare if I didn't match lions to lions and zebras to zebras. Again not directly related to my disability but I'm 57 deep and still trying to pull a real like out of my... umm hat.

58) Back to nada

59) Been a another week, but the reality is; there is nothing I truly like about being handicapped. I promised 75 and have produced nothing so I'll keep thinking.

60) I like dogs. I had a great German Shorthaired Pointer named Diego. He never asked me what was wrong with me, never got embarrassed in public with me, just showed me unconditional affection. I gave him up for a girl who wouldn't be seen in public with me, told me I couldn't go on walks with her, eventually slept in another room… bottom line is that dog had far more compassion than that… oops, almost used a derogatory dog term, but it is really unfair to female dogs to refer to her as an equal.

61) 61! I feel real bad readers, I know I indicated 75 and here we are at 61. I asked for some assistance but the only suggestion I received was a telepathic demand to go do something that I believe may be physically impossible. I'll take a nap and see what I can come up with.

62) After sleeping and sleeping and sleeping you can call me Rip Van Winkle, but don't call me gay. My single status has nothing to do with sexual preference (I love the girls) but that appears to have been beyond my brother in laws comprehension. Countless holidays I was lucky enough to endure his ridicule and his gay accusations. I shouldn't be overly surprised as his IQ is only slightly inferior to the turkey, ham or 4th of July Oscar Meyer wiener placed on the table. I can say that until number 62, I had never stooped to his level but I'm not even sure he can read, so I think I'm safe. "Hey I represent that remark", says brother in law! No you idiot, you RESENT it!

63) I like Sun, 3 wheeled recumbent cycles. I don't own one, I'd like to, but lack of funds prevents it. I think it would be good exercise for me but my income barely affords

an internet connection to look at computer pictures of them.

64) Again, I know I'm reaching and irritating you to come up with ONE legitimate "like" but I can assure you I'm trying my best.

65) Oh how's this one? I have a tremendous tolerance to pain, isolation and compassion for others in similar life struggles. I have a far greater sense of empathy for any ones struggles in life regardless of predicament. Believe that to be a character issue, but more than likely a direct result of understanding.

66) SIXTY SIX! Less than 10 to go and still a big fat nothing. I've spanned many months and years trying to establish a quality like, but I continue to encounter a lack of benefit or positive attribute.

67) I like swimming. I understand the benefits of swimming and every

sense childhood I've enjoyed being in, on or around the water. I do however and rather obviously lack a swimming pool. I also despise the stares and comments I tend to receive while in a swim suit amongst the masses, so as much as I wish to swim and maintain some strength, it is not even an annual event to publically utilize a pool.

68) I like my lifelong friends Andy, Keith and Kenny. They have occasionally treated me with kid gloves when it was warranted, but I got beat down, I got wacked, I got put in my place when the situation called for it. I always appreciated the Mac's for their kindness towards me and I'll never forget Mr. Marty's delivery of oranges, eggs and sausage when hard times were present. A special acknowledgement is needed to the Guppies for an extraordinary gift which I foolishly squandered. Hindsight is 20/20 they say and

provided the knowledge of hindsight, I would never have given Diego up! It may be a simplicity, but decent, good people do decent, good things. I truly like I have been afforded some decent, good people in my life even if they do now live a 1000 miles from me.

69) I like sarcasm. However this could be a sarcastic response. I do concede it has nothing to do with being handicapped but I'm still drawing blanks.

70) 何も

71) רבד םוש

72) لا شيء

73) I like that I'm narrowing in on 75. It has been mental torture all this time I've spent trying to conjure up a "like" and although I'm disappointed in my lack of "likes", I am certain I did try my best to come up with some.

74) I liked the 4th and 6th grades. I was probably at my physical peek and began to go downhill from there. I couldn't run fast but I could still run and play. Had some great classmates, no worries in the world other than how foul the mood my father was in. I biked, skateboarded, swam and kept up with my peers fairly well. Still not a handicap "like" but about as close as I can get.

75) I like this is the last time I have to try and come up with something, because it just is not going to happen. There's simply nothing I like about being bent, broken, mocked, abused and looked upon as sub-human. Treated as if I lacked human feelings, equal rights, opportunities, employment or the desire for companionship. For those of you that read this and think I should just suck it up and enjoy life as it is, well you are indeed entitled to your opinions.

The fact I have a handicap doesn't provide for an absence of my own opinions and thoughts. And I think my opinion is precisely how I feel. I hate it, I will never accept it, I will never be happy imprisoned in this body. After nearly 50 years of being me, I'm rather certain I have a pretty good idea of what it's like to live my life. I have the experience and qualifications to render opinions on what I like and hate about being handicapped. Sorry if you read this book expecting inspirational script. I know some that have handicaps and are quite content, pleased to be themselves. I am not one of those people. But I do hope you found some humor, some understanding and some preferred etiquette when it comes to dealing with handicap people. Adios amigos!

Dedicated to my friend Matt who like me grew up with muscular dystrophy. Unlike myself and much to my envy, Matt always seemed comfortable in his own skin. We never discussed things like that, we were too busy arguing supremacy; Plant or Daltrey? Bonham or Moon? Beatles or Stones? Who looked better that day Diane or Barbara? How many seconds it would take Josh or Aaron to beat up Bigfoot?

He died peacefully in his sleep some years back but was fortunate enough to have accomplished his goal of being a disc jockey, father to 2 outstanding kids and countless personal goals.

www.ingramcontent.com/pod-product-compliance
Lightning Source LLC
Chambersburg PA
CBHW060008300526
45794CB00003B/1142